# The Best Secrets of Natural Remedies

### BY LINDSEY P

## The Ultimate Guide to Natural Remedies to Prevent and Cure Illnesses, Cold and Flu for Your Family

## 2nd Edition

# Table of Contents

# Introduction

I want to thank you and congratulate you for purchasing the book, "The Best Secrets of Natural Remedies: The Ultimate Guide to Natural Remedies to Prevent and Cure Illnesses, Cold and Flu for Your Family".

This book contains proven steps and strategies on how to treat and prevent illnesses, cold and flu using natural remedies. You will learn and discover from the information presented in this book:

- The three secrets that your family doctor may not have told you about natural remedies and conventional treatment

- How some of your kitchen staple ingredients are actually as effective as drug-based medicines in curing and preventing diseases and how they are much safer to use with no negative side effects

- Why you need to have a strong immune system to resist and prevent cold and flu and other common ailments and how you can build your immunity from illnesses.

The information you will find from this book are to increase your awareness and understanding of the power of natural remedies to treat and prevent illnesses.

This e-book does not intend to replace any medication you are taking for your ailment or disease. You must never stop any medication you or your family members are currently taking without discussing it with your physician. Use the information herein as your guide to make better choices and decisions.

Thanks again for purchasing this book. I hope you enjoy it!

# Chapter 1. Natural Remedies Secrets Your Doctor Did Not Tell You

Do you know that your body has the natural ability to heal itself? As such, you do not have to depend on prescription or over-the-counter (OTC) medicines all the time to treat and prevent an illness of any member in the family.

Here are three (3) natural remedies secrets that your doctor may not have told you.

- Natural remedies work with your body systems to prevent and cure illnesses, cold, and flu. What they do is to activate your systems ability to fight and defend your body against the causes of these illnesses with no side effects.

  Medicines, on the other hand, may bring you faster results. However, they usually relieve the symptoms and therefore results are often temporary.

  Doctors will never tell you that all medicines contain toxic ingredients in varying levels. This is why medicines have side effects ranging from common, mild to severe, and life threatening.

- While medicines are convenient, natural remedies such as herbs and vitamins are often the solution to prevent and cure diseases. The thing is, most doctors are wired to prescribe drug-based medicines, and seldom, if they do, will they discuss with their patients the potency of natural remedies to cure and prevent sickness.

Would it be illogical to think that doctors and drug makers co-exist? The prescription drug industry is a big business. It is obvious that drug makers would not give up their industry for natural remedies, even if there were substantial proof that the latter is more beneficial in preventing and curing diseases.

For their part, doctors will not prescribe natural remedies over drug-based medicines for two reasons:

- Their focus is not to prevent diseases, but to treat them. The simple answer is that they earn more from treatment of diseases than from their prevention.

  Following logic, the more patients they have to treat, the higher their income. This is not to mention the incentives from the pharmaceutical industry.

- They lack the support from legislators, who in turn, are greatly influenced by the pharmaceutical industry. Funds for training and studies usually come from drug makers.

  Therefore, it is a difficult road ahead for any doctor to pursue training or research on the healing (preventive and curative) powers of natural remedies.

- There is no patent for natural remedies. From a business perspective, any solution that is not patentable is not a wise investment.

Hence, pharmaceuticals will not invest or put their money on research, studies, and tests that will document the proof and validate the efficacy and safety of natural remedies to prevent and cure illnesses, colds, and flu.

Natural cures are not big businesses. In order for drug makers to use ingredients from nature and patent it, they have to change its structure by mixing it with synthetic substances. The introduction on unnatural ingredients is what makes drug-based medicines toxic to the body.

The thing is, these natural substances from nature that are not patentable, are the ones that work best with the body to prevent and cure diseases, including those that are life threatening. Their best advantage is that they bring permanent results without side effects even with long-term treatment.

# Chapter 2. Natural Ingredients That Can Prevent and Cure Illnesses

Nature has blessed humanity with natural ingredients that can help the body heal and recover from illnesses. The best treatment and cure is always prevention. In instances requiring treatment, these ingredients also work, especially when the illness is not a medical emergency.

In this chapter, you will discover five (5) of the best natural ingredients that can prevent and cure illnesses. You must have them readily available in your home. You may use these ingredients as first aid or as natural solution to protect your body against ailments and diseases.

## i. Garlic

This natural ingredient is a versatile home remedy that can work as:

- ✓ Anti-bacterial
- ✓ Anti-fungal
- ✓ Anti-viral

Dr. Joseph Mercola of Mercola.com recommends daily consumption of one (1) medium-sized clove of fresh garlic. Crush the garlic before you take it with water, or you may also use it as an added ingredient to your juice.

## What It Can Do to Treat and Prevent Illnesses

Here are the things garlic can do in the prevention and treatment of illnesses:

- It is an effective prevention against cancer. Garlic contains allicin, a natural substance that gives it its distinct albeit strong flavor and smell. The reaction from crushing the garlic allows allicin to penetrate, inhibit, and kill cancer cells in the body.

- As a heart-friendly ingredient, garlic promotes healthy heart by doing these things:

  - Improves the numbers of your total cholesterol
  - Restores the normal balance between your LDL (bad cholesterol) and HDL (good cholesterol)
  - Prevents the hardening of the arteries, a condition that leads to heart attack and stroke
  - Lowers high blood pressure
  - It has the potential to reverse cardiovascular diseases

- Garlic can act as an anti-cancer agent.
  - The sulfides present with high garlic consumption have the ability to reduce the risk of colorectal cancer by as much as 50%
  - Daily consumption of garlic can also lower the risk of stomach cancer

- It is your natural defense against infections
  - It fights infection without killing the good bacteria in the body. It is safe to consume.

Antibiotics have the tendency to become less effective with the body developing resistance to it with prolonged or repeat use.
- o It can also clear your body of infections from fungi and parasites.

- Garlic can prevent and treat the following:
  - o Insect bites such as from mosquitoes and ticks
  - o Digestive disorders
  - o Colds and flu
  - o Sinusitis
  - o Liver disease
  - o Circulatory disorders
  - o Ulcers
  - o Insomnia
  - o Arthritis
  - o Asthma

## ii. Ginger

This herb is popular not only as a kitchen staple, but also as a natural medicine because of its healing properties. Since centuries ago, this herb has been used to treat various illnesses. It has extremely high levels of antioxidants, specifically phytochemicals, a natural substance in plants that can heal the body.

## What It Can Do to Treat and Prevent Illnesses

Here are the benefits you can get from ginger as a natural

remedy:

- Ginger is a very good source of Vitamin C that can strengthen your immune system.

  It is also rich in minerals such as copper, magnesium, manganese, and potassium. The immune system is the body's shield against diseases.

- It can detoxify your intestinal tract. This will prevent gastrointestinal disorders such as but not limited to the following: upset stomach, gas, and diarrhea.

- If you are nauseated or vomiting, ginger is your effective natural solution to get rid of nausea and to stop your vomiting. This is because, according to Dr. Mercola, ginger stimulates good saliva flow.

  Further, Dr. Mercola considers ginger as more effective than Dramamine, an OTC medication, in curing motion sickness. Ginger also works excellently and safely in relieving morning sickness and pain.

- It can work to stimulate fever for the treatment of and recovery from certain diseases and ailments (from simple to life threatening) such as the following :
  o Colds and flu
  o Lyme disease
  o Malaria
  o Cancer

  This is because fever is a mechanism for the body to heal, inhibit and/or eliminate pathogens (bacteria, fungi, parasites, viruses, and other infectious agents).

- It is an extremely effective anti-inflammatory agent. Ginger can treat and prevent unnecessary inflammation, the root of many diseases. It encourages the healing properties of inflammation.

  Chronic inflammation, on the other hand, results with the following health conditions, and are therefore treatable with ginger:

  o Arthritis
  o Periodontitis
  o Atherosclerosis (hardening or thickening of the artery walls)
  o Hay fever
  o Gallbladder Carcinoma ( an unusual type of cancer)

### iii. (Extra) Virgin Coconut Oil (VCO)

Start to replace your usual cooking oil in your kitchen with (extra) virgin coconut oil, and you will see how your health will improve. The body will benefit from the fats you can receive from coconut oil, which is an excellent source of your caloric energy. This oil, unlike other oils, is heat resistance that preserves the oil's rich antioxidant content.

### What It Can Do to Treat and Prevent Illnesses

Here are just some of the ways you can use (extra) virgin

coconut oil as a powerful natural remedy for illnesses:

- Coconut oil contains lauric acid, the same natural substance present in a mother's milk. Lauric acid in coconut oil and breast milk transform into monolaurin upon consumption, the natural compound that strengthens the immune system.

  The immune system is the cornerstone of the body's defense against illnesses and diseases. It is impossible to enjoy good health condition without a strong immune system. It is both your shield and your weapon against pathogens.

- The fats present in coconut oil can actually help you burn more unnecessary fats in your body. Too much fat in the body can lead to a condition you know as obesity. This condition is a precursor to several ailments such as heart diseases, diabetes, high blood pressure, high cholesterol, infertility, and cancer.

  Coconut oil can help you get rid of your weight because the fats in coconut oil belong to the medium chain fatty acids or MCFAs, which your body immediately converts as consumable energy instead of reserved fat storage.

- Like garlic, it defends your body against bacteria, fungi, and viruses. You will have a better protection against infections caused by these pathogens when you include coconut oil in your diet.

  In fact, studies reveal that coconut oil has the ability to kill an extremely dangerous pathogen,

Staphylococcus Aureus that harms the skin and respiratory tract. It can also guard your body against yeast infection, as coconut oil kills Candida Albicans.

- It promotes good dental health. It inhibits the bacteria present in your mouth that cause tooth decay. Several studies also prove that coconut oil has properties that can eliminate the cause of mouth infections including oral thrush without any side effects.

You and your family can benefit much with the process called "oil pulling". This method involves swishing pure coconut oil in your mouth for a few minutes similar to gargling with mouthwash. In doing so, the coconut oil will pull toxins and pathogens to treat and prevent dental problems.

Oil pulling is not limited to promoting good dental health; it has other benefits such as the following:
  o Pain relief from headaches and migraines
  o Helps in the treatment of diabetes mellitus and asthma
  o Controls and prevents acne breakouts

- MCFAs in coconut oil work to improve the functions of the brain, especially those who have the mild form of Alzheimer's disease. The fatty acids supply the brain with necessary energy to boost its cognitive functions.

In people suffering from mild Alzheimer's, studies show that their brains are deficient in energy. This is because certain parts are not functioning well in using glucose to produce consumable energy.

What coconut oil does is to correct this deficiency. It sees to it that the brain receives adequate levels of energy converted from glucose. The result is an improvement in your mental function.

## iv. Apple Cider Vinegar (ACV)

The strongest potentials and capabilities of apple cider vinegar (ACV), according to Dr. Mercola, are in the treatment and prevention of Type 2 diabetes. Studies confirm that ACV can help lower high blood sugar, a condition that leads to diabetes.

## What It Can Do to Treat and Prevent Illnesses

While more research and studies are still necessary, ACV has already shown its potentials in treating and preventing the following illnesses:

- Insulin resistance – this is the condition where body cells are unable to respond to insulin. Since the body resists insulin and its functions, this leads to hyperglycemia or high blood sugar.

  In a study by the WebMD, results show that consumption of two (2) tablespoons of ACV before bedtime can correct blood sugar levels. The only side effect to ACV consumption to treat and prevent insulin resistance is weight loss.

- Seborrheic Dermatitis or Dandruff – is easily treatable and preventable with apple cider vinegar, according to the medical team of experts of the Dr. Oz television show.

  The acid content of ACV is what works to eliminate dandruff on your scalp. The vinegar changes your scalp's pH level, denying the dandruff the condition it needs to persist and thrive on your scalp.

  You just need a mixture of apple cider vinegar and water in equal parts. Spray the mixture on your scalp and hair, avoiding your eyes and ears. Cover your hair with towel and leave the ACV mixture on for up to an hour. Rinse your hair. You can ditch the family's anti-dandruff medication or shampoo, as ACV is a safer option.

- High Blood Cholesterol – experts at the WebMD acknowledges the potentials of ACV in treating and lowering high blood cholesterol. The acetic acid content of ACV is the one responsible for lowering LDL or bad cholesterol in the body.

  A study with rats as subject in 2006 revealed how apple cider vinegar can lower LDL and triglycerides effectively. A Japanese manufacturer of condiments conducted his own research and found that about .5 fluid oz. of ACV taken daily can lower bad cholesterol in human beings.

- Atherosclerosis – is the thickening of the artery walls. This results with clogged or narrowed blood passageway. If blood that carries oxygen is not able to circulate freely to the heart and the brain, the person with this condition is likely to suffer from either a heart attack or stroke.

  The reason for the thickening of the artery walls is plague build up from cholesterol deposits. Your natural solution to treat and prevent atherosclerosis is to add apple cider vinegar as part of your heart-friendly and healthy diet.

- Parasites – that pester your puppy or dog cannot win against ACV. Your pet is a family member that you should also protect against illnesses. A common cause of an illness in your pet is parasite bites and infection.

  Apple cider vinegar protects the skin of dogs from parasite bites and infection. You can apply the vinegar externally or internally. Spray the ACV-water solution on your pet's fur and skin, as the solution will work as an anti-parasite (flea, ticks, and mites) agent. You can also mix it with your pet's food to encourage good skin condition and good health.

## v. Onion

The healing and medicinal properties of onions date back in ancient times. Like garlic and ginger, onion is a kitchen staple and a common cooking ingredient. It is rich in properties and nutrients that promote good health. This includes the natural substance that gives onion its distinct albeit strong smell.

## What It Can Do to Treat and Prevent Illnesses

Consider these benefits from onions:

- High Polyphenol Content – onions are the seventh highest in polyphenol content, higher than garlic and ginger. Polyphenols shield the body against free radicals and related pathologies that can cause the following: cancer, heart ailments, and inflammatory diseases.

  It will be a pleasant surprise to you and to your family that this kitchen staple has higher polyphenols than commonly believed. It is also extremely rich in flavonoids and quercetin that work as anti-viral, anti-allergy, anti-inflammatory, anti-tumor, anti-platelet aside from its antioxidant activities according to the Department of Environmental and Molecular Toxicology of the Oregon State University.

- Anti-Cancer – studies reveal that consuming onions regularly can reduce your risk of certain types of cancer such as ovarian, colorectal, and laryngeal as well as breast, esophageal, and oral cancers.

  Dr. Fuhrman who recommends consumption of high nutrient density food considers onions and garlic as anti-cancer food. These two staple ingredients are rich in organosulfur compounds that can fight and prevent the growth of cancer cells in the body. To maximize your anti-cancer benefits from onions, consume it chopped or crushed.

- Heart-Friendly – the sulfur compounds present in onions can prevent the clotting of blood and can improve blood flow. These compounds also discourage blood platelets to form into a clump or mass that trigger cardiovascular diseases such as heart attack.

The antioxidant content of onions is also beneficial in lowering cholesterol, specifically bad cholesterol and triglycerides. Further, onions can improve the functions of your red blood cells such as transporting oxygen.

- Anti-Inflammatory – onions have nutrients and properties such as Onionin A (sulfur-containing compound) that can inhibit the activities of your white blood cells that result with unnecessary inflammation.

While inflammation protects the body from harmful stimuli such as bacteria, viruses, and fungi, unnecessary inflammation triggers chronic inflammatory diseases such as rheumatoid arthritis, type 1 diabetes, inflammatory bowel disease, and multiple sclerosis.

- Bone Health – studies show that the nutrients in onion can strengthen the bones and increase its density. Women who are into their menopausal stage can benefit much from including onions in their healthy diet. With increased bone density and stronger bones, there is lesser risk for osteoporosis and hip fracture.

To get the most benefits for bone health from onions, you should make it a point to consume it generously on a daily basis. When peeling onions, preserve as much of the outer layer as possible, as this is where the flavonoids are richest. Over peeling your onions can result with a loss of up to 70% of its polyphenol content including flavonoids, quercetin, and anthocyanin.

The key in maximizing your health benefits from these five (5) natural ingredients is to incorporate them with a healthy diet and exercise regimen.

# Chapter 3. Healing Through Nature's Elements

If you're a pragmatic, down-to-earth, no-nonsense person, you may be skeptical about healing with color, water, or seawater products. We don't claim that any therapy in this ebook will work for everybody, so of course, we don't know whether or not these will do anything for you, but they've all worked for somebody—actually a lot somebodies—or else they wouldn't be listed here.

## i. Using Colors to Remedy Illnesses

### What Color Therapy is

Color therapy is the use of color for physical, mental, and emotional healing. In some forms, color therapy is closely akin to light therapy but with the addition of specific colors.

### What Illnesses It Can Remedy

Physiological: Chronic pain, skin diseases, muscle aches, neuralgia, rheumatism, arthritis, migraine headache, jaundice, overweight, vision problems

Psychological: Stress, agitation, depression, lethargy, overeating, violent behavior

### What You Need

Colored paints, light fixtures with colored filters, or clothing in particular colors

## How Color Therapy Came About

We know that color therapy dates back at least as far back as Ancient Egypt. In that time, Egyptian priests built healing temples that contained separate rooms, each painted in one of the seven colors of the rainbow: red, orange, yellow, green, blue, indigo, and violet. A patient was placed in one of these rooms to heal. The room in which the patient was placed depended on the nature of the illness or injury.

The Ancient Greeks also built light temples that made use of color for healing. Pythagoras, the great Greek mathematician, was an early proponent of the therapeutic use of color. In the East, color was a component of health and healing in both the Chinese and Ayurvedic traditions.

People probably first noted the effects of color in the day and night cycles of their lives and in the changing seasons. The "day" colors red, orange, and yellow seemed energizing, while the "night" colors blue, indigo, and violet were calming and restorative.

*Color and the Life Process.* We perceive color when light enters our eyes and moves through neurological pathways to the brain. The cortex of the brain, the most "educated" part, knows the names of the colors, differentiates one from another, and reacts aesthetically to color. However, our more primitive midbrain also reacts to color instinctively and more out of reflex. The midbrain's reaction to color suggests that at some level color is involved in the whole life process.

Through animal studies, scientists have found that certain regions of the brain respond differently to different wavelengths of light (colors). This means that we may be able to influence various functions of the endocrine system with colored lights.

Ancient writings in Sanskrit tell us that long ago, Indian scholars were aware of this possibility. According to their theory, the body is composed of seven major energy centers known as chakras. Each chakra is located at the site of major endocrine glands. The chakras correspond to particular states of consciousness, and each is governed by a color.

Today, most scientists accept that colors can have psychological effects on human beings, but there is more controversy surrounding the physiological effects of color. A number of scientific studies support the premise that color can affect heart rate, blood pressure, and respiration rate. One study found that yellow light caused the greatest increase in these rates and black light the greatest decrease.

*Color and Healing.* Modern practitioners use blue light to treat neonatal jaundice and arthritis pain. Blinking red light has been found to be effective for treating many patients with migraine headaches. Other physicians use blue light for the same problem. Experts have found that bubble-gum pink is a color that calms and alleviates aggressive tendencies, so this color is used to paint the walls of jail cells, juvenile reformatories, mental institutions, and other locations where aggressive behavior is a problem. Because it has such a calming effect, bubble-gum pink (also called Baker-Miller pink) can also reduce the nervous tendency to snack in overeaters.

Red and blue lights may affect athletic performance. One study found that viewing red light gave athletes quick bursts of energy, whereas blue light produced a steadier level of energy.

## How to Perform Color Therapy

Color therapy is of two types: the use of pigments or dyes (as in wall colorings or clothing) and the use of colored lights. For DIYers, the use of colored lights should be confined to regular light bulbs with colored filters.

Want to change the way you feel through the colors of the clothing you wear? The chart below can help you choose the right color to create a certain mood:

Red: Strength, dynamism, courage

Yellow: Happiness, carefree attitude, ability to communicate

Green: Stability, feeling of abundance

Calm: Inner peace

Orange: Vibrancy, sexuality, self-esteem

Purple: Connection with higher purpose

Black: Self-effacement (some people say that black absorbs negativity and keeps it from touching the person.

White: Clarity, focus

If you want to use color in your home to advantage, try bright colors in rooms where you want to be stimulated and alert. Use shades of blue or green for the bedroom. Orange is said to stimulate the appetite, so you might want to put a little orange into your dining room and kitchen. Very dark colors are generally depressing, so you may want to stay away from dark brown, gray, and black.

Some people believe that the benefits of colors can be absorbed by water. If you want to try water treated in this way, fill a red glass pitcher with water and put it in a window where the sunlight strikes the glass. (The longer you leave the pitcher in the sun, the more of the red light is absorbed, according to proponents.) To get a greater boost in energy, use this water to make your morning beverage. You can do the same thing with a blue glass pitcher to prepare water for a calming effect. Use water treated with a blue light for a soothing drink before bed. Some health care practitioners report that they have successfully treated ulcers with water exposed to green light and constipation with yellow-charged light.

You can also use colored lights for healing. A plain lamp with various colored filters that can be changed is probably the easiest to use. The chart below lists some uses for various colored lights.

Red: Urticaria, eczema, circulation, vitality, energy, anemia, muscle contractions, rheumatism, arthritis

Orange: Asthma, respiratory disorders, cramps and spasms, digestion, general body normalizer, hiccups.

Yellow: Constipation, arthritis, promotes wakefulness

Green: General healing, balance, congestion

Blue-green: Stress, fever, inflammation

Turquoise: Headache, swelling, sunburn, itching, burns, skin toning

Blue: Fever, stress, high blood pressure, sore throat, insomnia, baldness

Indigo: Ear problems, eye strain, insomnia

Violet (this is violet-colored light, not ultraviolet light): Cramps, high blood pressure, bladder problems, neuralgia

Magenta: General stimulant, diuretic.

## ii. Simple Water Therapy for Healing

### What Water Therapy is

Water therapy, or hydrotherapy, is the internal or external use of hot or cold, fresh or mineral water for healing.

### What Illnesses It Can Remedy

Physiological: Muscle aches, sprains, arthritis, rheumatism, eczema, psoriasis, blood circulation, pain, inflammation, hemorrhoids, back pain, colds, flu, headache, infections, joint stiffness, overweight, sinus problems, wounds

Psychological: Stress, tension, insomnia, inability to concentrate, nervousness, phobias, smoking addiction

### What You Need

Depending upon the form of therapy, you may need a tub, pool, spa, whirlpool, or shower. You may also need wet cloths or towels, and you might like to add aromatic oils or herbs to your bath.

### How Water Therapy Came About

Water is essential to all forms of life, so it is not surprising that this wonderful refreshing fluid has been used for healing since the dawn of humankind. Ruins of nearly all ancient civilizations include some form of bath. Cretans, Egyptians, and Babylonians all soaked themselves for health and relaxation, and they practiced other forms of water therapy as well. So did the Hindus in long-ago India.

In the fifth century BC, the Greek physician Hippocrates

touted natural spring water for its healthful effects, and somewhat later another physician, Galen, developed a whole regimen of exercise massage and bathing for the sick.

Water therapy was popularized in Europe in the mid-19th century by a German priest, Father Sebastian Kneipp, who developed a cold water treatment that apparently cured his own tuberculosis. Father Kneipp's treatment, known as the "Kneipp Cure," later featured not only cold water, but sunshine, fresh air, and regular activity as well. The cure also included walking barefoot on the dew-moistened grass or snow, alternating between hot and cold baths, and warm wraps.

The Kneipp Cure was well-known in Europe for many years before it finally came to the United States in the early 1900s. Kneipp wrote several books about his treatment, the most famous of which was *Meine Weskur* ("My Water Cure").

Dr. John Harvey Kellogg was an American physician, surgeon, and inventor of medical devices. He was also a proponent of many forms of natural medicine, and in his sanitorium in Battle Creek, Michigan, he treated patients with hydrotherapy, diet, and other non-drug therapies. His book *Rational Hydrotherapy* became a model text on the subject.

Kneipp and Kellogg helped to make hydrotherapy known in the United States, but it had actually been practiced here all along. Native Americans built "sweat lodges" that were similar to saunas to cure disease. Healing herbs were often added for their aromatic vapors. After inhaling the vapors in the sweat lodge, the patient would go outside for a cold plunge into a nearby river or snowbank.

Hydrotherapy is probably as popular today as it has ever

been, although most people relaxing in a sauna or hot tub probably don't realize they're giving themselves a "treatment."

## How to Do Water Therapy

The ways in which you can use water as therapy are nearly limitless, and you probably already know most of them. Here's a quick list to jog your memory:

- Drink six to eight glasses of pure water daily. (Mineral water is fine.)

- Soak your feet in a tub of very warm water after a long day. Then quickly run cold water over them and give them a brisk rubdown.

- To ease tension, soak your whole body in a tub filled with warm water. Add your favorite herb or scented oil for a special treat.

- For relief of arthritis, soak in a hot tub (temperature no higher than 104° F) for no more than fifteen minutes. Put a cold washcloth on your head to prevent headache or congestion. Obviously, if you have a real "hot tub," you can use this instead, but don't exceed the time and temperature. (Hot tubs are not recommended for pregnant women or people with circulation problems, high blood pressure, nerve impairment, diabetes, or heart disease) After the hot bath, splash with cool or lukewarm water to normalize your blood vessels.

- Fill a basin or the wash bowl with very hot water, drape a towel over your head and inhale the steam. Add some herbs if you want to. This is a great skin treatment, and it can help clear your nasal passages if you have a cold or sinus congestion. Try adding some eucalyptus oil if congestion is your problem.

- Lie down and cover your eyes and forehead with a warm wet towel to banish stress and/or relieve a minor headache.

- Swim or do water exercises to keep yourself fit.

- Turn your shower on to needle-sharp or pulsating mode to massage aching muscles

- Try alternating between hot- and cold-water baths/showers or wet packs to soothe pain. Hot, then cold, baths are called contrast baths. They promote healing in a variety of conditions by causing the blood vessels to alternately dilate and contract. This sets the blood pumping and improves circulation. Start with four minutes of hot (104° F) water, then one minute of cold (59° F) water. Repeat the process five or six times.

- Relax (if you can) in a warm sitz bath to relieve the discomfort of hemorrhoids. (For a sitz bath, just put a few inches of water in the tub and sit with your feet flat so that your knees are raised.)

- Either a cold or warm sitz bath can help relieve the pain and swelling after childbirth.

- Having trouble falling asleep? Try a just-above-skin-temperature (about 100° F) bath just before bed. Soak for as long as a half hour, dry off, and go to bed immediately.

- Got a migraine? A hot shower followed by a cool one might help.

- Try using your feet to alleviate a cold or cure a sinus headache. Soaking your feet in a hot tub pulls blood from the head to the feet and may unclog your nasal passages.

## ii. Simple Water Therapy for Healing

### What Thalassotherapy is

Thalassotherapy is the therapeutic use of seawater or products derived from seawater.

### What Illnesses It Can Remedy

Physiological: Rheumatism, arthritis, skin diseases, metabolic imbalance, circulatory problems, cellulite

Psychological: Stress, tension

### What You Need

Seawater and/or products containing marine botanicals, such as seaweed and algae

### How Thalassotherapy Came About

From the Greek *thalassa*, meaning "sea," thalassotherapy really dates back to the first ocean bathers, whoever they may have been. The sea has always bewitched humankind. People have idolized it, feared it, frolicked in it, and lazed on its shores, but always they have respected its awesome power. From ancient times, people have looked to the sea for restoration and health. The Greeks, Romans, Cretans, Egyptians, and Babylonians built communal baths where they bathed in water brought from the sea. The Egyptians were fond of a vegetable known as a sea onion that grew near the shore. The sea onion was also used for medicinal purposes.

In the Orient, vegetables from the sea often grace the family table. From ancient times, Orientals have eaten various forms of seaweed and kelp, and they have used them for healing purposes.

In Victorian England, people flocked to the seashore for their holidays. At that time, hot and cold seawater baths were among the amenities offered by coastal resorts.

Although products from the sea have been used for healthful purposes for a long time, the term thalassotherapy is a relatively recent one. In 1869, a French physician coined the name for therapy that uses seawater and sea vegetables for a variety of treatments that include baths, facials, massages, body wraps, and cosmetic products. The French are still devotees of thalassotherapy; many French spas use piped-in seawater for their baths and showers, and personal-care products containing marine botanicals abound.

Sea plants and the water itself are rich in vitamins, amino acids, metalloids, and minerals. Proponents of thalassotherapy claim that these elements can be taken into the body through the skin to stimulate the body's own natural immune system, boost circulation and hasten the elimination of wastes and toxins. Interestingly, the salts in seawater and sea vegetables are very similar to those found in human blood serum. Some people feel that this suggests that humans had an aquatic ancestor or two. Others merely cite the resemblance as evidence for why thalassotherapy works.

### How to Do Thalassotherapy

Some spas and holistic health centers offer thalassotherapy treatments, but you don't have to live on the coast or fork out big bucks to see what thalassotherapy can do for you. There are a variety of personal-care products on the market that you can use at home. (If you use sea salt for cooking, you've already made a tiny entry into the field.)

Most of these products contain seaweed, a vegetable rich in iodine, calcium, magnesium, potassium, sulfur, sodium, trace elements, and vitamins A, D, and E. Believers say that seaweed conditions and nourishes hair and skin and helps them retain moisture. You can buy cleansers, masks, moisturizers, shampoos, lotions, bath salts (a popular product comes from the Dead Sea), shower products, slimming gels, and creams that purport to control cellulite. If you want to emulate a spa experience, you might also want to try a seaweed body wrap. Follow that with a Sea Mud Mineral Soak (Erno Laszlo), which instantly turns your bathwater a beautiful cerulean blue, and you'll be transported to the Mediterranean without ever leaving home!

Here's a partial list of the benefits of seaweed:

- Softens and soothes dry skin and makes it more supple and elastic

- Humps the skin so wrinkles are less visible

- Promotes cell division and regeneration

- Adds body, sheen, and softness to hair; controls dandruff

- Helps remove cellulite from the hips and thighs by releasing and eliminating toxins.

Oil of algae is another marine botanical that is said to have restorative powers. Massaged into the skin several times daily, it can control fungal skin infections, such an athlete's foot and fingernail fungus. Mothers also use it to prevent diaper rash and cradle cap in their babies.

# Chapter 4. Natural Remedies for Cold and Flu

Cold and flu are two of the most common ailments that can affect the whole family. As the saying goes, cold and flu never leave the house without one member passing it to the rest. The ailment can spread rapidly.

Understand that over-the-counter medicines for cold and flu are symptom reliever. Unless the symptoms bother you or any of your family members much, then you are better off taking the natural approach to treat and prevent the spread of cold and flu.

### i. Preventing the Spread

First, here is how to prevent the spread of cold and flu when a family member has it:

- Keep on reminding everyone in the family the necessity and importance of washing their hands often. Use water and soap, and in their absence, you may substitute with hand sanitizers.

  To wash hands the right way, follow these simple steps:

  1. Wet your hands up to your wrists with clean water.
  2. Apply the soap thoroughly to cover all parts of your hands including your wrists. Do a gentle

rubbing and massaging of your hands, palms, fingers, and wrists when applying the soap.
3. Rinse your hands and your wrists well.
4. Dry with a clean hand towel.

- Maintain good hygiene. The following are basic practices that every member of the family should do regularly:

  ✓ Take a bath every day.
  ✓ Keep your body dry and clean.
  ✓ Wash hands properly before you touch anything to prepare the meals, eat your meals, touch your body, and after touching anything including your pet or going to the bathroom.
  ✓ Be sure to clean your body and change your clothes before going to bed at night.
  ✓ Brush your teeth after every meal.
  ✓ Cover your mouth when yawning and most especially when coughing or sneezing, to prevent the quick spread of the cold and flu virus.

- Avoid sharing utensils, towels, and other personal items with any member that has the cold or the flu. The cold and flu virus can use these things as channels for transmission.

- Keep your home clean particularly common areas and things that are commonly touched such as doorknobs, water taps, and counters.

## ii. Strengthening the Immune System

A strong immune system is what you and the rest of your family members need to prevent cold and flu to visit or linger in your household. You do not have to spend much to build a strong defense system against cold and flu, as most remedies you already have in your home.

According to experts at the Harvard Medical School, the immune system's ability to function well depends on balance and harmony. While further research and studies are necessary to identify how the system works and what will keep the balance and harmony, there are measures that you can do to start boosting your immunity, especially against common ailments such as cold and flu.

These experts from Harvard recommend that you follow healthy living strategies that consist of the following:

- Eat a well-balanced and healthy diet comprising mostly of fruits and vegetables. The high nutrient density diet by Dr. Joel Fuhrman makes sense with this recommendation, as fruits and vegetables are the types of food that measure the highest in nutrient density.

  Here are the top 5 food types highest in nutrient density:

  1. Raw Leafy Green Vegetables, e.g. romaine lettuce, kale, and spinach - the darker the color of the veggies, the higher the density of its nutrients

2. Solid Greens, e.g. asparagus, bok choy, broccoli, celery, okra, and string beans among others – the best ways to consume these veggies are raw or steamed

3. Non-green and non-starchy veggies, e.g. mushrooms, onions, red and yellow peppers, tomatoes, and beets

4. Beans and legumes

5. Fresh fruits

Here are the best food items for immunity:

1. Kale
2. Arugula
3. Green lettuce/cabbage
4. Broccoli
5. Carrots /tomatoes
6. Garlic and onions
7. Mushrooms
8. Berries
9. Pomegranate
10. Seeds

- Increase your physical activity to lose unnecessary weight. You should prevent your body from storing fats by using more energy to burn calories. The key is to stay active. Move your body and avoid being a couch potato.

Moving your body through doing physical activities also helps to optimize the circulation of blood that carries oxygen and nutrients from food to the different parts in your body. Find the time to exercise, and do it consistently.

According to experts at Medline Plus, simple exercise routines can boost your immune system to fight bacteria, viruses, fungi, and other pathogens. Your consistent routine will also enable your body to fight off cold and flu easily.

What exercise can do to the body are the following:

- o Flushes out bacteria from the lungs and therefore this reduces your risk of cold and flu as well as other airborne ailments

- o Improves the functions of your white blood cells and antibodies to detect, warn, and protect your body against pathogens such as bacteria and viruses

- o Enables your immune system to fight infections effectively while slowing down the growth and spread of bacteria and viruses in the body

- o Delays the release of stress hormones that contribute to the risk and occurrence of illnesses

The combination of diet and exercise is your foundation for a strong immune system. To further boosts your immunity, the Harvard team of experts suggests the following:

- Avoid unhealthy vices such as smoking and excessive

drinking.

- See to it that you and other family members are within your recommended weight level, and start losing excess weight.
- Regulate blood pressure.
- Get enough sleep, rest, and relaxation. This allows your body to recover from stress and restore its normal functions.
- Lower your risks of infections by practicing good hygiene and washing your hands properly
- You and your family members should consult your physician at least twice a year whether you are sick or well.

## iii. Home Recipes to Treat Cold and Flu

To treat cold and flu when you or any member in the family has it, you may benefit from the following home remedies:

## Natural Cough Syrup

Cough is a common symptom of cold and flu. To stop cough, here is a better syrup solution that is natural and chemical-free:

- You will need the following ingredients: a cup of raw honey, about two to three tablespoons of lemon juice, and ¼ cup of warm drinking water.

- Mix the honey and lemon juice in a clean glass container. Slowly pour the warm water into the mixture.  Stir until all ingredients and well combined.

- Administer one to two teaspoons of the lemon honey syrup before bedtime.

## Chicken Soup for the Cold

Chicken soup is not only good for the soul; it literally heals your body from common cold and flu.  Science backs this up.

Here is a healthy recipe of chicken soup for the cold:

- You will need the following ingredients: chicken meat (preferably from free roaming chicken), egg noodles, spring onions, parsley, thyme, celery, carrots, salt and pepper for seasoning, chicken flavored cubes, water, and bay leaf.

- Combine the chicken meat, water, cubes, celery and thyme in a pot and bring it to a boil.  Remove the chicken, and throw away the celery.  Filter the broth to remove chicken fat.  Add some water and all the other ingredients save for the bay leaf.  Bring to a boil or until the noodled are ready.

- Add the chicken meat and the bay leaf.  Cook for another five (5) minutes.  Remove the bay leaf and prepare to serve the chicken soup.

## iv. Reminders

Keep in mind that while all the natural remedies have their

own individual benefits, they work best with a holistic approach.  For instance, even if you increase your consumption of onions if you are not following a healthy diet, you may not be able to see results.

It is also best that you consult with your physician not only when you or any of your members are not feeling well. Taking preventive measures against illnesses, cold and flu is always better and preferable than curing it.

# Chapter 5. Breathing Styles that Heal

Healthful breathing means deep breathing to bring plenty of oxygen into the body and to get rid of carbon dioxide and other waste products. Oxygen is a tonic for the whole body. A healthy dose of oxygen to the brain stimulates mental faculties; infusing the bloodstream with oxygen revitalizes cells and builds up a store of energy. The more energy we have, the better we can go about our daily tasks and the better we can fight off diseases.

## i. Pursed-lip Breathing

### What Pursed-Lip Breathing is

Pursed-lip breathing is a technique that helps those who are chronically short of breath breathe easier during physical activity.

### What Illnesses It Can Remedy

Physiological: Asthma, bronchitis, emphysema, other chronic obstructive pulmonary diseases

### How the Idea of Pursed-Lip Breathing Came About

Most people with respiratory ailments can neither inhale nor exhale deeply enough. Shallow breathing causes these people to run out of air during even light exertion like walking up a flight of stairs. Often people with breathing difficulties have airways that are constricted or filled with mucus. To help alleviate these problems, respiratory-care specialists began to teach pursed-lip breathing to their patients. Today pursed-lip breathing is taught in many respiratory-care facilities and hospitals. Use of the technique probably evolved simultaneously in various facilities rather than being developed by one individual.

## How to Do Pursed-lip Breathing

Pursed-lip breathing is very simple. Just inhale through your nose. Pucker your lips as if you are going to kiss someone, and then exhale slowly through your mouth. That's all there is to it. The reason this works is that this type of exhalation builds up pressure in the airways, which helps to keep them open. If you've got breathing problems, try this technique the next time you walk up a flight of stairs and see if you aren't less breathless than usual when you get to the top. Even if you don't normally have breathing problems, you probably get winded during vigorous aerobic activity. Try pursed-lip breathing top help you keep the pace.

## ii. Diaphragmatic Breathing

## What Diaphragmatic Breathing is

Diaphragmatic (pronounced dye-a-fra-mat-ic) breathing is just what it sounds like: breathing from the diaphragm rather than from the upper chest. Diaphragmatic breathing provides better air intake and strengthens the lungs; it is especially good for people with breathing problems.

## What Illnesses It Can Remedy

Diaphragmatic breathing can help remedy asthma, bronchitis, emphysema, and other chronic obstructive pulmonary diseases.

## What You Need

You will need a comfortable chair with a straight back and a mat, rug, or carpeted floor to lie on to do the strengthening exercises.

## How the Idea of Diaphragmatic Breathing Came About

People who breathe without thinking about it usually breathe from the chest only. If you have respiratory problems, chest breathing may not be deep enough to keep you from becoming short of breath upon even mild exertion. Respiratory care specialists sought a way to help people with this problem learn to pull more air into their lungs and thus to inhale and exhale more deeply. One solution—borrowed in large measure from yoga—is diaphragmatic breathing.

Today diaphragmatic breathing is often taught in the respiratory care departments of local community hospitals.

## How to Do Diaphragmatic Breathing

Diaphragmatic breathing is just what it sounds like: breathing from the diaphragm (the muscular band that separates the cavity containing your lungs from the abdominal cavity). Diaphragmatic breathing is easy once you get the hang of it, but it may seem unnatural at first. Normally, when someone asks us to take a deep breath, we expand the chest and suck in the gut. On exhalation, we allow the gut to relax and distend. If you want to do diaphragmatic breathing, forget that. Instead *push out* the gut as you inhale, and then pull it in as you exhale slowly.

Try to develop a rhythmic motion, like a wave rising and falling. To see if you're doing it right, put your fingers under your rib cage. Your finish should lift as the abdomen rises.

Diaphragmatic breathing takes a little practice, but it's worth learning. You can combine diaphragmatic and pursed-lip breathing by inhaling from the diaphragm and exhaling through pursed lips. It may also help to develop a rhythm that coordinates with your physical activity. While walking, for example, inhale then take three steps as you exhale. Repeat.

*Exercises to Strengthen the Diaphragm*: If your diaphragm is very weak, you may have to work on strengthening it before you can get the maximum benefit from diaphragmatic breathing. Doing the diaphragmatic breathing itself will make your diaphragm stronger, but if you want to get results faster, try these exercises:

1.  Lie on the floor with a small pillow or folded towel under your head and shoulders. Clasp your hands behind your knees but keep your feet flat on the floor.

    - Inhale.

    - Exhale while bringing your elbows up toward your ears as if you were trying to touch your elbows together.

    - Inhale as you move your arms back to the floor.

    - Repeat the sequence.

2.  Lie on the floor with knees bent, feet flat. Put your hands just below your ribcage.

    - Inhale.

    - Exhale and press down with your hands.

    - Relax your hands and inhale again.

    - Repeat the sequence.

### iii. Pranayama: The Indian Style

## What Pranayama is

Pranayama (pronounced prah-nah-yah'-mah) is the science of correct breathing as developed by ancient Indian yogis.

## What Illnesses It Can Remedy

Physiological: Asthma, bronchitis, emphysema, poor complexion, colds, sinus problems, weak intestinal and abdominal muscles

Psychological: Anxiety, stress, lethargy, smoking cessation

## What You Need

If you choose to sit or lie down for the breathing exercises, you will need a comfortable chair with a straight back and/or a mat or carpeted floor.

## How Pranayama Came About

In Sanskrit, the ancient language of India, *prana* means "life force," and *yama* means "control." Therefore, pranayama translates into "control of the life force." For thousands of years, yogis and other scholars and philosophers of the East have taught that there is a primal creative force—prana—that permeates the universe. Yogis believe that prana is the sustainer of all life, whether plant, animal, or human. When prana is present, the being is alive; when it is absent, the being is dead.

According to this philosophy, the more prana a person has, the more fully alive and healthy he or she will be. People can learn to increase their intake of prana, and they can store it in their bodies. The key to doing this is through correct breathing which should be combined with proper living habits and use of the mind for maximum benefit.

Centuries ago, yogis observed that the animals with the shallowest, quickest breathing were more nervous than other creatures, and they had shorter life span. The mouse is one of those animals. On the other hand, elephants and turtles breathe long and slowly. These animals are calm, and they live a very long time. It was from these observations that the yogis developed their breathing exercises.

## How to Perform Pranayama

Pranayama is an integral part of yoga, but we have included the breathing techniques separately here because you can use them on their own even if you do not wish to learn the whole discipline. Two important breathing techniques are the cleansing breath and complete breath.

Sitting cross-legged is the traditional way to perform yoga breathing and, but you may sit in a chair, stand, or even lie down for some exercises if that is more comfortable.

*The Cleansing Breath.* To perform the cleansing breath, which is sometimes known as bellows breath or runner's breath:

- Sit upright in a comfortable position.

- Inhale through your nose, but not deeply—about a third of a lungful of air is about right—while at the same time expanding your abdomen outward as far as you can.

- Quickly and vigorously contract your abdomen while forcefully expelling all the air from your lungs through your nostrils. This quick exhalation should be very vigorous. (It's similar to the effect of being unexpectedly punched in the stomach.)

- Expand your abdomen outward again and inhale through your nostrils.

- Repeat the vigorous exhalation through your nostrils.

Remember, all the breathing is done through your nose. Each cleansing breath is one relaxed inhalation and one forceful exhalation. Each should be completed in one or two seconds.

Because the exhalation is so forceful, the cleansing breath removes some of the pollution and other impurities that we breathe into our lungs. It is an excellent early morning wake-up technique as well as a quick refresher any time during the day when the mind is fatigued.

Along with the other yogic breathing techniques, the cleansing breath may help you to overcome the smoking habit, but you will probably have to practice it patiently for some time in order to have this effect. People who have used the cleansing breath to help them stop smoking say that once they've become accustomed to flushing out pollution and other impurities with the cleansing breath, they have no desire to inhale them again by smoking.

*The Complete Breath*: To perform the complete breath:

- Sit in a comfortable position breathing normally.

- Pull in your abdomen and exhale through your nose until you've expelled all the air from your lungs.

- Push your abdomen outward while at the same time inhaling slowly and rhythmically through the nose.

- Still inhaling smoothly, pull your abdomen in slowly and expand your chest by pulling your breastbone forward and expanding your rib cage.

- Begin exhaling, and relax your shoulders and chest.

- When all the air has been expelled, you have finished one complete breath.

The entire procedure should be rhythmic and wavelike.

You will probably have to predict the complete breath a number of times before you develop the proper rhythm. The complete breath can be performed while standing, sitting cross-legged, lying down, or sitting in an ordinary chair.

The complete breath has a wonderfully calming and relaxing effect, and it helps strengthen the abdominal and diaphragmatic muscles. The increased oxygen available during the exercise may induce the release of endorphins, which could account for its remarkable effect on stress.

# Chapter 6. Healing with Your Arts and Hobbies

Art, music, and other hobbies are wonderful activities that you can lose yourself in and forget about the cares of the day, but only if you find pleasure in doing them. These are not activities you should take up because somebody tells you they're good for you. If you don't enjoy them, they'll only make you frustrated and angry that you're wasting your time. Find something else.

## i. Using Visual Arts to Promote Well-being

### What Art Therapy is

Art therapy is the therapeutic use of the visual arts to promote physical and emotional healing. Professional art therapists use the shapes and pictures that their clients make as a means of nonverbal communication that can lead to a better understanding of the client's behavior. This type of treatment is not a do-it-yourself project, however, and it is outside the scope of this ebook. Self-help with art therapy as described here refers simply to the emotional and/or physical benefit that a person can derive on his or her own from creating artistic projects.

### What Illnesses It Can Remedy

Physiological: Headache, stroke, arthritis, rheumatism

Psychological: Alcoholism, drug abuse, emotional problems, learning disabilities, tension, stress

## What You Need

The equipment and materials depend upon the art medium you choose. Costs can range from a few dollars for a sketch pad and pencils or charcoal to a hefty outlay for a kiln, potter's wheel, clay, glazes, and other paraphernalia for ceramic work. If you want to try something that costs a lot for equipment and supplies, it's best to take a course first to see if you really like the activity before spending quite a lot just to outfit yourself.

## How the Idea of Art Therapy Came About

Long before there were written words, there was art. Humankind's desire for artistic expression goes back at least to the time of the cavemen. Throughout history, standards in beauty have changed with the times, but art remains a powerful means of self-expression that mirrors the view of the world.

We can still appreciate the great works of art from earlier times because they have been lovingly preserved for their beauty and significance, but surely there was a caveman who was all thumbs who nevertheless daubed away at the walls of his cave, uncaring that his bison was only a blob with legs. Some early Roman must have taken up a hammer and chisel and hacked away at a piece of marble vainly attempting to carve out a recognizable human head. Great works of art end up in galleries and in public plazas; art works created by lesser mortals almost never meet the public eye.

Why, then, do people whose works fall woefully short of meeting current standards of beauty continue to carve, paint, sculpt, and throw clay against a wheel? Because it makes them feel good.

The origins of art therapy as a profession date back to the

last century when some scholars began to take an interest in the psychological aspect of art. As they pursued this line of thinking, they came to realize that creating art met some inner need in many people.

Later mental health professionals recognized that, although their patients often could not express their feelings in words, they could do so nonverbally through art. Art became a tool through which professionals could learn things about their patients.

## How to Perform Art Therapy

Professional art therapists are trained to recognize the significance of symbols and patterns, and they have a background in normal and abnormal behavior and skills in intervention methods. Professional art therapy is one form of psychological treatment, which is sometimes used alone but often in conjunction with other treatment methods. Obviously, you can't treat yourself with this kind of therapy; you have to consult a professional.

You can, however, use art to relax, reduce tension, vent hostility and aggression, and in some cases, improve motor skills. You don't have to have any talent, you only have to find what you do therapeutic and enjoyable. Think of it as a hobby with health benefits.

You don't even have to do art on a regular basis. Mad at your husband? Draw a picture of him with horns and a tail and big ugly fangs. Vent your anger on paper, and you may be surprised to find it melting away.

The form of art that you choose depends upon what appeals to you, your pocketbook, and the kinds of benefit that you'd like to get. Working with clay can provide needed exercise for arthritic hands. Painting big, bold designs on huge canvases can provide a sense of freedom for people who feel boxed in by too many responsibilities. Feel distracted and unable to concentrate? Try something detailed that demands close attention.

If you're intrigued by doing some kind of art but don't quite know what you'd like to try, you might want to experiment by taking some classes. In most communities, you can find classes in painting, drawing, and ceramics that are geared to amateurs. Try your local community college or high school (Many high schools offer "lighted schoolhouse" programs where you can use the facilities of the art and ceramics departments after hours under the supervision of a professional.). Ceramic supply stores often offer classes too.

You may not become another Michelangelo or be discovered by a famous art critic, but that doesn't matter. If art provides therapeutic benefits for you, then never mind that one eye is higher than the other on that face you drew. Picasso's work looked funny to a lot of people too.

## ii. Listening to Music to Aid in Healing

### What Music Therapy is

Music therapy involves either listening to music or playing an instrument for its therapeutic value.

### What Illnesses It Can Remedy

Physiological: Asthma, hypertension, migraine, intrauterine and post-partum infant growth stimulation, pain, trauma recovery, stroke recovery, senile dementia, Alzheimer's disease, physical movement limitations

Psychological: Insomnia, anxiety, depression, stress,

hyperkinesis, autism, learning and communication disabilities

## What You Need

*Listening:* Equipment for playing recorded music

*Playing*: Musical instrument(s) of your choice

## How the Idea of Music Therapy Came About

Ancient. The first use of music was utilitarian, not aesthetic, and vocal, not instrumental. Early practitioners of magic sought to imitate sounds of nature, believing that "like affects like." That is, sounds approximating those of one's surroundings were avenues for communicating with and modifying forces thought to influence natural phenomena, physical and spiritual well-being, and behavior. Imitation led to organization, deliberate and purposeful repetition, and creation of sound messages meant to convey the wishes, direction, and power of the practitioner relative to his or her environment.

Unlike other arts, music was considered by early societies to be divine in origin. As such, it was an important intercessional tool for use as a palliative for simple discomfort, a potent curative for demonic possession, or an alternative "voice" for communicating directly with deities. The Greeks and Chinese found dinnertime melodies an affective aid to digestion. Native American and African shamans drummed and chanted away evil spirit. And the Christian church from its beginning regarded some music as divine, other music as evil or pagan. Just as David relieved the Israelite King Saul's melancholy and uncontrollable fits of rage with the playing of his harp, contemporary physicians and therapists use music in the treatment of chronic and acute mental, emotional, and physical disorders. The mathematical precision inherent in music lends itself well to therapeutic application.

## How to Do Music Therapy

Self-directed music therapy is possible whenever and wherever you can establish a comfortable site free of interfering sensory distractions. Your own bed, an easy chair, or a grassy hillside—almost any location is suitable as long as it does not compete with the music. Of greater importance than setting, however, is the selection of music for listening. Although taste in music is highly subjective, there are certain guidelines that are helpful in creating specific therapeutic environments.

*Technique for Listening*: Set aside a time block of approximately an hour when you know you will not be disturbed. Choose a comfortable site for sitting or reclining. Whether you use a headset or conventional speakers is a matter of choice; again, your comfort is the most important consideration. Wear loose clothing. If it suits your mood, dim or cover any bright light sources, including the sun. It is best to activate the continuous loop option, if there is any, for your recordings so that you can keep the music playing and not break the mood created by the music.

A normal heartbeat ranges from sixty to eighty beats per minute. You might want to check your pulse before and after your listening sessions, perhaps even chart it, in order to monitor the effectiveness of your therapy. It is possible to slow your heartbeat and actually lower your blood pressure, at least temporarily, by quietly listening to music with a beat somewhat slower than your heartbeat. Because popular music usually has a beat considerably faster than sixty beats per minute, you will have to choose your selections carefully. Try the *Venus* portion of Holst's *The Planets*, the first movement of Ravel's *Mother Goose Suite*, or Bach's Brandenburg Concerto No. 4.

On the other hand, just as music can be effective in slowing bodily functions, it is also very useful for setting a pace for physical activity. For instance, if you are doing aerobic exercises, walking, or taking part in some other conditioning regimen, some selections of march music or other spirited music will help you maintain an even steady pattern for your repetitive movements. Music is effective in teaching rhythm, particularly with children who may require patterning exercises or autistic persons who seem most comfortable in a regulated environment.

Those persons who have difficulty with motor skills may find the fingering of guitar strings, flute fingerholes, or piano keys beneficial.

The ability of music to create a therapeutic atmosphere is well known. Some musical selections have a calming effect while others may be useful for mood elevating. Recognition of personal taste is essential in choosing music intended for psychological reaction The piped-in "elevator music" so prevalent in office buildings is intended to produce a restful, pleasant ambiance. To some listeners, however, it has exactly the opposite effect, setting their teeth on edge and making them irritable.

If you enjoy playing a musical instrument, this can also be therapeutic. Try soothing melodies to relax, lively ones to lighten your mood. Something rousing or difficult to play can drain away anger. Do you play an instrument that you can attack with vigor, like the piano or drums? By all means, give it a workout and let your tensions go. Learning a new piece can help you temporarily forget a vexing problem, but it's probably the wrong choice if you're playing to calm down. In that case, it's better to choose something that you can play effortlessly so you can let the flow of the music work its magic.

Some people make music part of their daily lives. If you're one of those who listens appreciatively and often throughout the day, you're probably already getting an incidental therapeutic benefit, but you may want to set aside a time just for listening (or playing).

Most people who seldom listen to music don't dislike it; they just don't think about it much. If you're one of these, try adding music to your life. In this modern age, it's just a click away, and you may find it's just the ticket to get rid of a pounding headache or lull you to sleep at the end of a busy day.

### iii. Getting in Contact with A Pet to Promote Healing

### What Pet Therapy is

Pet therapy uses contact with a pet to promote emotional and psychological healing.

### What Illnesses It Can Remedy

Physiological: Hypertension, overweight, cardiovascular benefits (e.g. from walking a dog)

Psychological: Depression, stress, tension, insomnia, feelings of isolation.

### What You Need

The equipment you need depends upon the type of pet you choose. Most pet needs are obvious, but if you're uncertain as to what you might need to keep a given type of pet, check with a veterinarian.

## How the Idea of Pet Therapy Came About

Wolves became the first domestic dogs, when early people decided they could tame these animals to help them with their work. In the beginning, dogs were not pets as we know them today; they worked for a living, principally as herders and hunters. However, through close contact, people and animals grew to trust and have affection for one another.

Cats have had a rocky road throughout history. In ancient Egypt, they were pampered and revered, but later, during the Middle Ages, when people got hysterical about witchcraft, cats were thought to be witches' "familiars," and they were often tortured and burned.

Since ancient times, people have kept birds in cages to enjoy their colorful plumage and cheerful songs. Medieval hunters often trained falcons to hunt prey. Although falcons weren't pets, there was close contact between man and bird.

Over the years, people began to keep more and more animals simply as pets. Today, in the United States alone, people own roughly sixty million dogs, fifty million cats, forty-five million fish, and eight million birds, not to mention all the rats, hamster, lizards, turtles, and other creatures that people might call pets.

Most pets are cherished members of the family, but it is only recently that researchers have discovered that pets provide health benefits for their owners. In an important study, investigators interviewed ninety-six people who were hospitalized for serious heart problems. One of the questions on the survey was whether or not they had pets. In a follow-up a year later, eighteen people had died. Twenty-eight percent of those who didn't have pets had died, whereas only six percent of those who did have pets had died. So Fido or Fluffy may be more than a friend; your pet could be a lifesaver.

Today pet therapy is a recognized form of treatment. Pets are often brought into nursing homes, hospitals, and even prisons for their healing effect.

## How to Use Pet Therapy

If you feel alone, depressed, or stressed out, you might want to consider a pet. Bonding with a dog or cat can help you feel less isolated, especially if you live alone. Remember, though, that a pet requires care, so don't get one unless you're willing to devote the time necessary.

When deciding what type of pet to get, consider your circumstances. A large dog, for example, might make you feel secure, but if you live in an apartment, a sheepdog probably isn't the pet for you. Big dogs require plenty of exercise whereas a few turns around the block may already be enough for a Chihuahua.

Cats make good pets for city dwellers, but you might also want to consider birds or fish. Watching fish swim lazily about their aquarium can be a very relaxing experience.

On the other hand, if you have the space and need to get more exercise, a big dog can be just the ticket. Dogs give you a reason to walk, and you and your pet can spend many pleasurable hours exploring your neighborhood on foot.

Before you get any pet, check with a veterinarian to find out the requirements of the particular animal you're considering. Some dogs get terribly lonely when left alone all day. If you work, take that into consideration. You might want to think about a cat instead or even a dog *and* a cat to keep each other company. Unless you have very little room, two pets aren't much more trouble than one, and you'll have twice as much companionship.

Remember that having a pet is good therapy only if you're fond of animals. If you don't like them, you're likely to have more stress by acquiring a pet, but if cozying up to a kitten sounds like just what the doctor ordered, it may truly be.

# Conclusion

Thank you again for purchasing this book!

I hope this book was able to help you to discover the secrets of natural remedies as your solution to treat and prevent common illnesses such as cold and flu.

Nature has gifted humanity with all the means to prevent and treat illnesses such as cold and flu. It is just a matter of finding what works best for your body as well as that of your family members. There is no one size fits all remedy, as each body is unique and will respond differently from treatments, whether natural or conventional.

You have learned from this eBook that natural ingredients can work like drug-based medicines in treating and preventing diseases. It just so happen that humanity is used to taking drug-based medicines especially when their doctors prescribe them. However, all drug-based medicines contain toxic ingredients, the reason they typically come with negative side effects.

If the illness is not an emergency that requires medical intervention, it is best to start developing the habit of using natural remedies for treatment and prevention. This will save you and your family from adverse effects of drug-based medicines (e.g. developing resistance to the drug and increasing the dosage, mild to serious complications).

Most of the ingredients that you need are already in your home, such as garlic, ginger, onions, virgin coconut oil, and apple cider vinegar. You will also need to improve the quality of your diet to include ingredients and food that will boost your immune system. Cold and flu do not stand a chance with a strong immune system.

The next step is to explore further the potentials and abilities of natural remedies in reversing diseases, and eliminating the need for medication. There is so much to learn and discover about the power of nature in healing the body.

Finally, if you enjoyed this book, please take the time to share your thoughts and post a review on Amazon. We do our best to reach out to readers and provide the best value we can. Your positive review will help us achieve that. It'd be greatly appreciated!

Thank you and good luck!

# Check Out My Other Books

Below you'll find some of my other popular books that are popular on Amazon and Kindle as well. Simply click on the links below to check them out. Alternatively, you can visit my author page on Amazon to see other work done by me.

Coconut Oil for Easy Weight Loss: A Step by Step Guide for Using Virgin Coconut Oil for Quick and Easy Weight Loss

http://www.amazon.com/Coconut-Oil-Easy-Weight-Loss-ebook/dp/B00JG8H8DE

Superfoods that Kickstart Your Weight Loss Learn How to Use 30 Superfoods to Boost Weight Loss, Immunity and to Live a Healthier Lifestyle

http://www.amazon.com/Superfoods-that-Kickstart-Your-Weight-ebook/dp/B00JNAPM9M

Carrier Oils for Beginners: Discover the Characteristics and Beauty and Health Benefits of Carrier Oils For mixing Aromatherapy Essential Oils

http://www.amazon.com/Carrier-Oils-Beginners-Characteristics-Aromatherapy-ebook/dp/B00K88GI2S

Natural Homemade Cleaning Recipes For Beginners: Essential Oil Recipes For Household Cleaning, Laundry & Toxic Free Living http://www.amazon.com/Natural-Homemade-Cleaning-Recipes-Beginners-ebook/dp/B00K87UBQI

The Best Secrets of Natural Remedies: The Ultimate Guide to Natural Remedies to Prevent and Cure Illnesses, Cold and Flu for Your Family

http://www.amazon.com/Best-Secrets-Natural-Remedies-Illnesses-ebook/dp/B00JNDCOCM

The Hypothyroidism Handbook:An Everyday Guide to Natural Solutions of living with Hypothyroidism including increased energy, lasting weight loss, and general well-being

http://www.amazon.com/Hypothyroidism-Handbook-Solutions-including-increased-ebook/dp/B00JNIGIV0

The Hyperthyroidism Handbook: An Everyday Guide to Natural Solutions of Living with Hyperthyroidism including Weight Gain, Increased Energy and General Well-being

http://www.amazon.com/Hyperthyroidism-Handbook-Solutions-including-Hypothyroidism-ebook/dp/B00JOHU5SM

Essential Oils & Weight Loss for Beginners: Ultimate Guide to Losing Weight, Increasing Energy, Balancing Metabolism & Appetite Using Essential Oils & Aromatherapy

http://www.amazon.com/Essential-Oils-Weight-Loss-Beginners-ebook/dp/B00JOFOWP6

Top Essential Oil Recipes: A Recipe Guide Of Natural, Non-Toxic Aromatherapy & Essential Oils for Healing Common Ailments, Beauty, Stress & Anxiety

http://www.amazon.com/Top-Essential-Oil-Recipes-Aromatherapy-ebook/dp/B00JY434E2

Soap Making For Beginners: A Guide to Making Natural Homemade Soaps from Scratch, Includes Recipes and Step by Step Processes for Making Soaps

http://www.amazon.com/Soap-Making-Beginners-Homemade-Processes-ebook/dp/B00JYKH75I

Body Butters For Beginners: Proven Secrets To Making All Natural Body Butters For Rejuvenating And Hydrating Your Skin

http://www.amazon.com/Body-Butters-Beginners-Rejuvenating-Hydrating-ebook/dp/B00K6LVV6A

Apple Cider Vinegar For Beginners: Proven Secrets Using Apple Cider Vinegar For Health, Weight Loss, and Skin Care

http://www.amazon.com/Apple-Cider-Vinegar-Beginners-Aromatherapy-ebook/dp/B00K6YY6HI

Homemade Body Scrubs & Masks For Beginners: 50 Proven All Natural, Easy Recipes For Body & Facial Masks To Exfoliate Nourish, & Care For Your Skin

http://www.amazon.com/Homemade-Body-Scrubs-Masks-Beginners-ebook/dp/B00K79D4SY

Essential Oils Box Set #1: Essential Oils & Weight Loss For Beginners (Ultimate Guide to Losing Weight, Increasing Energy, Balancing Metabolism & Appetite Using Essential Oils & Aromatherapy) + Top Essential Oil Recipes (A Recipe Guide of Natural, Non-Toxic Aromatherapy & Essential Oils for Healing Common Ailments, Beauty, Stress & Anxiety)

http://www.amazon.com/ESSENTIAL-OILS-BOX-SET-Aromatherapy-ebook/dp/B00K7Q8HRK

Essential Oils Box Set #2: Essential Oils & Weight Loss For Beginners (Ultimate Guide to Losing Weight, Increasing Energy, Balancing Metabolism & Appetite Using Essential Oils & Aromatherapy) + Top Essential Oil Recipes (A Recipe Guide of Natural, Non-Toxic Aromatherapy & Essential Oils for Healing Common Ailments, Beauty, Stress & Anxiety)

http://www.amazon.com/ESSENTIAL-OILS-BOX-SET-Aromatherapy-ebook/dp/B00K7Q8HRK

Box Set#3: Coconut Oil for Easy Weight Loss(A Step by Step Guide for Using Virgin Coconut Oil for Quick and Easy Weight Loss) + Apple Cider Vinegar(Proven Secrets Using Apple Cider Vinegar for Health, Weight Loss, and Skin Care)

http://www.amazon.com/Box-Set-Beginners-Aromatherapy-Essential-ebook/dp/B00K9TEGUW

Box Set #4: Body butters For Beginners(Proven Secrets To Making All Natural Body Butters For Rejuvenating And Hydrating Your Skin) & Top Essential Oil Recipes: A Recipe Guide Of Natural, Non-Toxic Aromatherapy & Essential Oils for Healing Common Ailments, Beauty, Stress & Anxiety http://www.amazon.com/Box-Set-Butters-Beginners-Essential-ebook/dp/B00KA02F4Y

Box Set #5: Soap Making For Beginners(A Guide to Making Natural Homemade Soaps from Scratch, Includes Recipes and Step by Step Processes for Making Soaps) + Homemade Body Scrubs & Masks For Beginners(50 Proven All Natural, Easy Recipes For Body Scrub & Facial Masks To Efoliate, Nourish, & Care For Your Skin)

http://www.amazon.com/Box-Set-Beginners-Homemade-Recipes-ebook/dp/B00K9U3I2I

Box Set #6: Body Butters for Beginners (Proven Secrets To Making All Natural Body Butters For Rejuvenating And Hydrating Your Skin) +Homemade Body Scrubs & Masks For Beginners(50 Proven All Natural, Easy Recipes For Body Scrub & Facial Masks To Exfoliate, Nourish, & Care For Your Skin)

http://www.amazon.com/Box-Set-Beginners-Exfoliating-Moisturizing-ebook/dp/B00K9U3Y4O

Box Set #7: TOP ESSENTIAL OILS(A Recipe Guide Of Natural, Non-Toxic Aromatherapy & Essential Oils For Healing, Common Ailments, Beauty, Stress & Anxiety) & THE BEST SECRETS OF NATURAL REMEDIES(The Ultimate Guide to Natural Remedies to Prevent and Cure Illnesses, Cold and Flu for Your Family)

http://www.amazon.com/BOX-SET-Essential-Recipes-Remedies-ebook/dp/B00K9WPMQG

Box Set #8: NATURAL HOMEMADE CLEANING RECIPES FOR BEGINNERS (Essential Oil Recipes for Household Cleaning, Laundry & Toxic Free Living) + TOP ESSENTIAL OILS(A Recipe Guide Of Natural, Non-Toxic Aromatherapy & Essential Oils For Healing, Common Ailments, Beauty, Stress & Anxiety)

http://www.amazon.com/BOX-SET-Beginners-Essential-Aromatherapy-ebook/dp/B00KAMNGBS

Box Set #9: Essential Oils & Weight Loss for Beginners (Ultimate Guide to Losing Weight, Increasing Energy, Balancing Metabolism & Appetite Using Essential Oils & Aromatherapy) + Carrier Oils for Beginners (Discover the Characteristics and Beauty and Health Benefits of Carrier Oils for Mixing Aromatherapy Essential Oils)

http://www.amazon.com/BOX-SET-Essential-Beginners-Aromatherapy-ebook/dp/B00KAODL6Q

BOX SET #10: THE HYPERTHYROIDISM HANDBOOK (An Everyday Guide to Natural Solutions of Living with Hyperthyroidism including Weight Gain, Increased Energy and General Well-being) + THE HYPOTHYROIDISM HANDBOOK (Everyday Guide to Natural Solutions of Living With Hypothyroidism Including Increased Energy, Lasting Weight Loss, and General Well-Being)

http://www.amazon.com/BOX-SET-10-Hyperthyroidism-Hypothyroidism-ebook/dp/B00KAKMSBY

BOX SET #11: CARRIER OILS FOR BEGINNERS (Discover the Characteristics and Beauty and Health Benefits of Carrier

Oils for Mixing Aromatherapy Essential Oils) + Essential Oils & Aromatherapy for Beginners (Secrets to Beauty, Health and Weight Loss Using Proven Essential Oil and Aromatherapy Recipes

http://www.amazon.com/BOX-SET-Beginners-Essential-Aromatherapy-ebook/dp/B00KAONEQ8


BOX SET 12: ESSENTIAL OILS & WEIGHT LOSS FOR BEGINNERS: (Ultimate Guide to Losing Weight, Increasing Energy, Balancing Metabolism & Appetite Using Essential Oils & Aromatherapy) + TOP ESSENTIAL OIL RECIPES (A Recipe Guide of Natural, Non-Toxic Aromatherapy & Essential Oils for Healing Common Ailments, Beauty, Stress & Anxiety) + CARRIER OILS FOR BEGINNERS (Discover the Characteristics & Beauty & Health Benefits of Carrier Oils for Mixing Aromatherapy Essential Oils) + ESSENTIAL OILS & AROMATHERAPY FOR BEGINNERS (Secrets to Beauty & weight Loss Using Proven Essential Oil & Aromatherapy Recipes) + NATURAL HOMEMADE CLEANING RECIPES FOR BEGINNERS (Essential Oil Recipes for Household Cleaning, Laundry & Toxic Free Living)

http://www.amazon.com/BOX-SET-12-Essential-Aromatherapy-ebook/dp/B00KCBCHE4


BOX SET #13: SUPERFOODS THAT KICKSTART YOUR WEIGHT LOSS (Learn How to Use 30 Superfoods to Boost Weight Loss, Immunity and to Live a Healthier Lifestyle) + ESSENTIAL OILS & AROMATHERAPY FOR BEGINNERS (Secrets to Beauty, Health and Weight Loss Using Proven Essential Oil and Aromatherapy Recipes) + BODY BUTTERS

FOR BEGINNERS (Proven Secrets To Making All Natural Body Butters For Rejuvenating And Hydrating Your Skin) + SOAP MAKING FOR BEGINNERS (A Guide to Making Natural Homemade Soaps from Scratch, Includes Recipes and Step by Step Processes for Making Soaps) + HOMEMADE BODY SCRUBS FOR BEGINNERS (50 Proven All Natural, Easy Recipes For Body Scrub & Facial Masks To Exfoliate, Nourish, & Care For Your Skin)

http://www.amazon.com/BOX-SET-Superfoods-Kickstart-Aromatherapy-ebook/dp/B00KC8G6DK/

BOX SET 14: Essential Oils & Weight Loss for Beginners (Ultimate Guide to Losing Weight, Increasing Energy, Balancing Metabolism & Appetite Using Essential Oils & Aromatherapy) + Apple Cider Vinegar for Beginners (Proven Secrets Using Apple Cider Vinegar for Health, Weight Loss, and Skin Care) + Body Butters For Beginners (Proven Secrets To Making All Natural Body Butters For Rejuvenating And Hydrating Your Skin) + Homemade Body Scrubs & Masks for Beginners (50 Proven All Natural, Easy Recipes for Body Scrub & Facial Masks to Exfoliate, Nourish, & Care for Your Skin) + Coconut Oil for Easy Weight Loss (A Step by Step Guide for Using Virgin Coconut Oil for Quick and Easy Weight Loss)

http://www.amazon.com/BOX-SET-Essential-Beginners-Aromatherapy-ebook/dp/B00KEDO68U

If the links do not work, for whatever reason, you can simply search for these titles on the Amazon website to find them.